Praise for *Unveil the Wounded Self...*

From the beginning, Jan's class, which focused on moving through and beyond a difficult experience, felt hopeful. With each writing we took another significant step toward deep healing. Jan brings to her teaching rich, relevant experiences from her own life and work, and she always was supportive and encouraging in her assignments and feedback. She shared with us valuable tools and resources to help us continue healing after the class is over.

—SUSAN, TEXAS

Jan Marquart's class, *Unveil the Wounded Self—Write to Heal*, provided me with the opportunity to start writing honestly and in a loving atmosphere about my trauma. It came at the right time for me; the journaling exercises and the healing tools provided a strong and efficient background which allowed me to put words on the unbearable and slowly but surely start embarking on my long healing journey. I highly recommend it.

—SABRINA, BORDEAUX, FRANCE

I recently took the *Unveil the Wounded Self – Write to Heal* course with Jan Marquart. Jan guided me through the 6 writing assignments, and more importantly helped me over the humps and bumps of a struggle over which I had been beating myself up for many years (I thought only about 10 years, but it came out, through the process of Unveil the Wounded Self, that it was much longer than that!). I'm not going to tell you there weren't painful moments during those 6 weeks; there were (though, fewer in number than the hopeful ones!). And Jan was there to accompany me through whatever wall I hit. There was always light at the end of the tunnel…I never thought a 6-week course could get me through something I had been challenged by for so long. I decided to work with Jan because I thought to myself, "I've tried everything else! I have nothing to lose!"

Not only did I not lose, I won—thanks to Jan and her unique combination of knowledge, insight and guidance. I recommend this course highly!

—BARBARA, USA

ALSO BY JAN MARQUART

Books for Adults

Write to Heal
The Mindful Writer, Still the Mind, Free the Pen
The Basket Weaver, a Novel
Kate's Way, a Novel
Echoes from the Womb, a Book for Daughters
Voices from the Land
The Breath of Dawn, a Journey of Everyday Blessings
How to Write from Your Heart (booklet)
How to Write Your Own Memoir (booklet)
A Manual on How to Deal with a Bully in the Workplace
Cracked Open, a Book of Poems
A Writer's Wisdom
Available at www.JanMarquart.com

Books for Children

Can You Find My Love? Children's theme-based book series:
Book 1: Seasons
Book 2: Things to Do Outside
Book 3: Why We Need Rain
Book 4: Things with Wheels
Book 5: Families
Book 6: Bugs
Book 7: In The Sea
Book 8: Morning
Book 9: On Your Head
Book 10: Babies
Available at www.CanYouFindMyLove.com

Unveil the Wounded Self

A Guided Journal for PTSD Sufferers

Unveil the Wounded Self

A Guided Journal for PTSD Sufferers

Jan Marquart LCSW

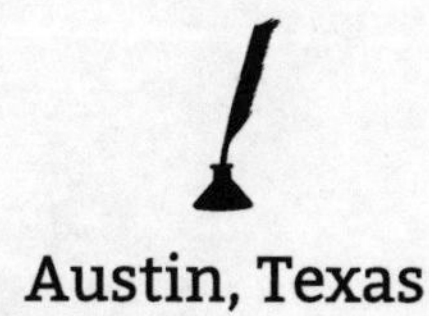

Austin, Texas

Jan Marquart LCSW
www.JanMarquart.com
www.janmarquartlcsw.wordpress.com

ISBN: 978-0-9973308-4-7

Designed by:
Janice St. Marie
Santa Fe, NM
janicestmarie@qwestoffice.net

This guided journal is dedicated, with hope,
to all those who suffer from PTSD and Complex PTSD
and who believe there is no way out of their darkness,
anxiety, depression, or dysfunctional behavior.

Acknowledgment

I'd like to thank Janice St. Marie, designer and friend, for helping me bring this important book to publication. I appreciate her creative ideas, unrelenting support, and help every step of the way. It is always a pleasure to work with her.

I can shake off everything as I write;
my sorrows disappear, my courage is reborn.

—Anne Frank
from *The Diary of a Young Girl*

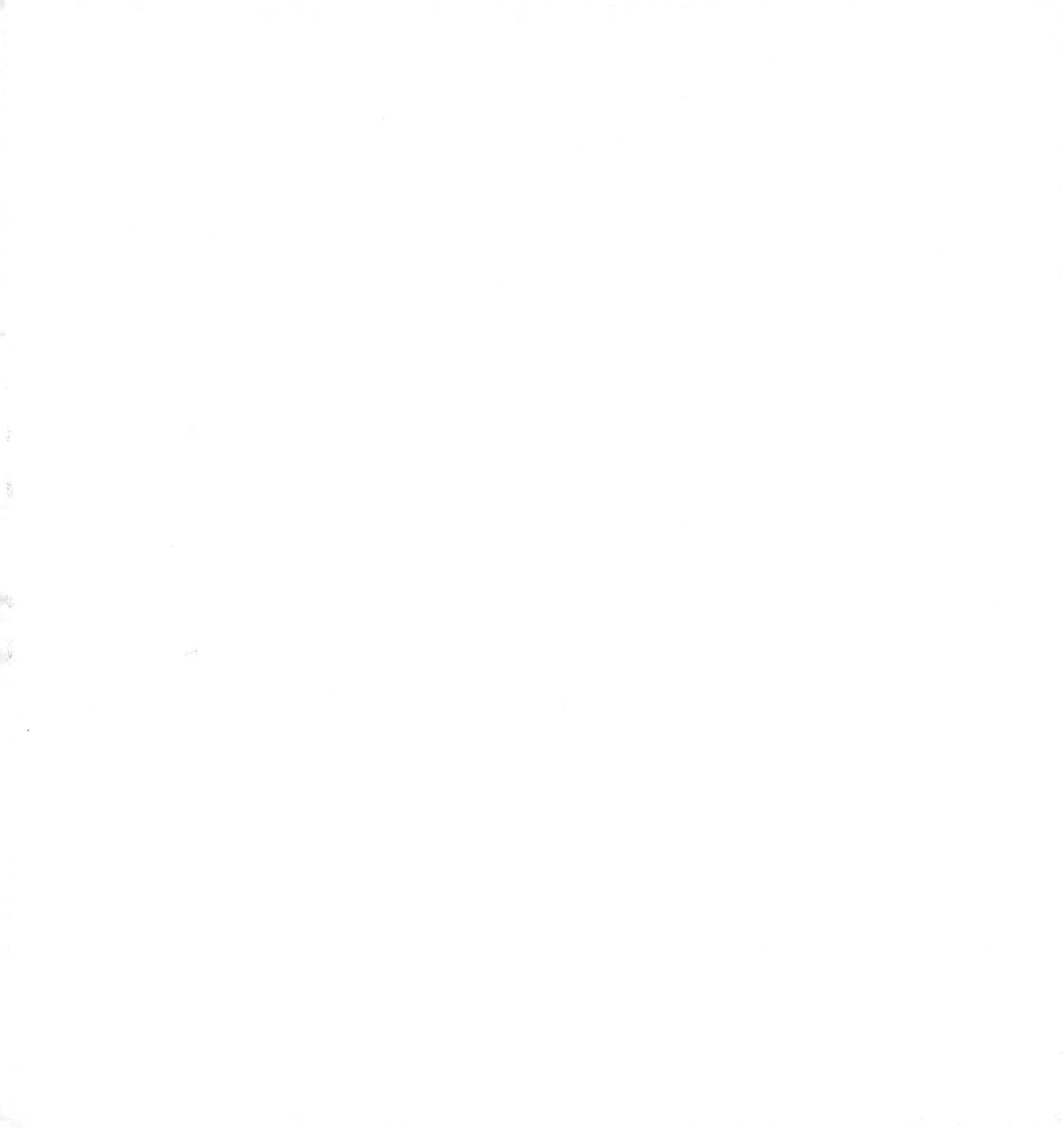

CONTENTS

The Physics of Emotions

You need only claim the events of your life to make yourself yours.
When you truly possess all you have been and done,
which may take some time, you are fierce with reality.

—Florida Scott Maxell
from *The Measure of My Days*

This journal is designed to help you overcome your traumatic experiences and get your life stabilized. In it you will find a 6-week writing course to help you uproot the traumatic event that happened to you, how you experienced it, and what to do about it. Before starting the process, review the List of Ideas for Calming Your Nervous System and please use them when writing excites or triggers distress. If distress erupts and you cannot calm yourself, please call a therapist or sponsor and talk it out. Completing these six steps will help you uproot the cause of trauma and help you control its symptoms.

Let's start with emotions. They do not stand alone but follow a certain pattern.

thoughts/beliefs → emotions → behaviors

To uncover, discover, and recover from trauma you must address all three elements. By realigning all three, you bring your life into a healthier balance.

What are emotions? Emotions are movements of inner energy that you experience all day long. You can start the day out with one emotion and end the day with another. Why is that? Because emotions are in direct correlation to all experiences of daily functioning. Emotional energy exists whether you like it or not. I call this inner movement the physics of emotions because that inner movement of energy is constantly changing and is always giving you information about what you are experiencing in every second. Emotions are not random. They are your internal messengers.

Thoughts/beliefs determine what emotion you feel and traumatic events wind up changing thoughts/beliefs simply because what has happened to you has fragmented life as you know it. Nothing in your internal world is the same anymore. In other words, you feel an emotion based on its thought/belief. Normally, you cannot think, "What a great day" and feel depressed. PTSD, however, is complicated. It is, I believe, a soul wound because whatever happened to cause trauma has gone about as deep as pain can go. Internally, PTSD causes a tornado of chaos. When the way you adapt to what happened is dysfunctional, those adaptive behaviors become symptoms of unresolved fragmentation. This is when you find yourself feeling 'broken.' See how the three elements, thoughts/beliefs> emotions>behavior are essentially one movement of cause and effect?

Think of flicking a group of marbles on a table. It might look as if the marbles are moving in a random motion around the room, but they are not. They are moving according to velocity, force, and gravity - the laws of physics. Imagine that each marble is one of your emotions. See the process? Your emotions will change according to what has impacted them, how hard they were flicked by your finger and how fast they traveled across the room.

When an event occurs, you cannot help but react. We are wired to react. Everything is in constant motion. It is the law of physics. Change cannot be avoided. Events change how you think, feel, and behave. All three have to change in order to accommodate what just happened. And when we can't change to accommodate what happened, in either our thoughts/beliefs, emotions, or behavior, for whatever reason, we are seriously impacted. And when the event causes such drastic changes that you cannot regain a healthy balance, you feel traumatized. Your reactions are not random any more than marbles moving across the table are. Some marbles will roll faster across the table, some slower, and some might fall to the floor, depending upon how hard you flicked them. Some of your experiences will flick you harder than others. Trauma will inflict shock, fragmented thinking, racing thoughts, anxiety, inner chaos, panic, numbness, sleeplessness, flashbacks, and abnormal behavioral reactions. Your body stress will increase. Illness may follow. Stress and illness go hand in hand. Over 90% of general physician office appointments are directly related to stress.

When you try to deny your emotions, push them away, or ignore them, they will only cause more stress. Rebalancing yourself after a trauma will not happen on its own. No one likes the dysfunction of everyday life that a traumatic event or events bring, however, only after the authenticity of what happened is confronted, acknowledged, and claimed for what it meant to you to have experienced it, can a functional life be restored.

Trauma shocks reality out of proportion. There are two types of trauma: PTSD and Complex PTSD. Complex PTSD is long-standing traumatization. Many mental health disorders apply to Complex PTSD. Passive/aggressive individuals are clear examples of this. People who are passive/aggressive are afraid of being angry, often due to witnessing and feeling fear of parental rage and strong control as children. As a result, their fear of being authentic creates a wound of loss disallowing a healthy expression of their own anger for fear they will be harmed by the raging parent. They withhold being authentic. Their behavior acts out anger in a sneaky, sometimes dangerous way. Bipolar, major depressive disorder, dissociative disorders and other significant mental health disorders can be led back to childhood trauma that remain unresolved. You know the story about the man who has a hard day and comes home and kicks the dog. Holding in emotions only serves to create other problems, i.e., illness and/or psychological disorders.

I once had a fabulous secretary. One morning I awoke to a bright, sunny, and warm day. It was glorious. I was in a great mood. When I got to work my secretary had tinfoil over all the windows darkening her small office. I asked her why she covered her windows on such a beautiful day. She said she felt pressure to be happy when it was sunny and she wasn't. Her way of adapting was to cover the windows and block the sun. As her story unfolded she revealed that she had been repeatedly raped by her father as a young girl. Sunny days only served to remind her of how unhappy and depressed she was and she'd have flash-backs of what happened to her. Her emotions of guilt and shame for not feeling the way 'normal' people felt were enormous. Her deep wounds were the loss of innocence, betrayal, and fear of vulnerability. These deep wounds changed her behavior in order to find a way to accommodate her pain. Covering the windows helped her in the moment but offered no healing for the deep trauma she had experienced by repeated acts of rape by her father. Trauma always reveals itself, somehow, in some way. Trust that your soul will always show you where you need healing.

There is an enormous amount of grief with traumatic experiences. Try to hold down your grief and what happens? Don't you feel the pain worsen? The healthy reaction to grief is crying but many people don't allow themselves the healing process of crying. Let yourself cry. It is an important part of healing. Crying allows your body to release the emotional energy of loss.

A powerful way to release toxic emotions, thoughts, and gain understanding of your behavior is to write. Writing is the language of the heart. When you write in your journal you can witness how your mind thinks, how your body feels and its emotions, and how to assess your behavior. Grief in trauma involves unmet desires, losses, failed dreams. When you take claim of what happened to you, you can restore and transform aspects of blocked pain.

Through writing you allow yourself the process of elasticity. What that means in the language of physics, is that something has an ability to resist a distorting influence or stress and return to its original form after the stress is removed. When you write, you help release and remove the toxic emotions of trauma that have distorted your thoughts, emotions, and behaviors. You then have the ability to be restored once the toxic trauma has been removed. Because you have a consciousness and inanimate objects do not (as in the marbles), you will raise to a healthier level of consciousness simply because by becoming more aware and assimilating your experiences into wisdom, you develop into another stage of relating to your life. You will never be able to remove what happened, but you will be able to grow through it. This is a process.

Many cultures have rituals and values to honor the emotional life of its people. In Egypt parents are expected to grieve for seven years after the loss of a child. In Hispanic cultures the Day of the Dead is a day to connect with deceased loved ones by cooking their favorite recipes. Indians have a three-day period called Ramadan to honor their deceased. But the Western world expects grief and shock to be time-limited. America is quite antiseptic and sterile when it comes to the mess emotions create in ordinary life. "Get control of yourself," is something Americans say a lot when people are upset, even traumatized. Then they call a physician for medication to avoid shame from having emotions upset the people around them. This philosophy is close to insane because it denies what we can't deny. The authentic message from your inner being about how you feel during tough times, *is* your mental health. This state is not something to be ashamed of; it is a declaration of your inner human integrity. We are wired to be emotional when we are impacted by life's events.

Studies show that writing diminishes depression, anxiety, even physical pain. Studies also show that when you write what you feel 20 minutes before sleep, sleep improves. Physical injuries heal faster when you write about the emotions involved in the injury. Writing helps clear emotional toxins and that can only serve for good.

PTSD and Complex PTSD assault your very soul. They are deep wounds.

You cannot see this energy but you feel it, you know it, you express it in a myriad of ways so that others see it. Perhaps your spouse tells you about your behavior and your boss tells you about your poor attitude. To write these experiences will not give you back your old life, but writing will put you on a path to re-create a life you want. To re-create a healthy life from this point requires a new narrative, one that develops new beliefs, emotions, and behaviors. Then you are on fertile ground to rebuild another foundation for well-being.

Twelve-step programs are replete with individuals who handled grief with alcohol, street drugs, pot, and prescription pain killers. Becoming an addict or abuser of substances does not cure emotional distress, it just gives temporary relief and tricks the mind to believe that, for the moment, all is well when, in fact, you are worse for it. You cannot exist as a human being without emotions. Here are some of the emotions you can feel on a daily basis:

Aggression
Anxiety
Apologetic
Arrogant
Angry
Bashful
Blissful
Bored
Cautious
Confident
Depressed
Determined
Disappointed
Disgusted
Ecstatic
Enraged
Envious
Exasperated
Exhausted
Frightened
Frustrated
Grief
Guilt
Happy
Horrified
Hurt
Hysterical
Indifferent
Interested
Jealous
Joyful
Lonely
Miserable
Negative
Obstinate
Optimistic
Paranoid
Perplexed
Puzzled
Regretful
Relieved
Remorseful
Sad
Satisfied
Shocked
Smug
Surly
Surprised
Suspicious
Sympathetic
Withdrawn

When you experience anything, you take it in non-verbally which means your body feels it first in the way of energy coming at you before you even get a chance to think about it. This energetic impact makes you feel an emotion or variety of emotions. In order to understand what happened and how your body registered the impact your mind structures it into thoughts/beliefs. This structure is the power of language.

Western culture demands that you get over emotional pain quickly by taking medication. The pharmaceutic market is replete with medications to help you get over messy emotions, however, medications only give you a reprieve from emotional distress by suppressing the symptom. When it comes to uprooting the reason for the distressful emotion, medications fall short. Medication is not designed to heal; it is designed to stifle symptoms. For a headache, Excedrin, which suppresses symptoms of head pain, might be all anyone needs. In the same light, those suffering from severe anxiety and depression will benefit from an anti-depressant or anxiolytic, but those medications still only suppress emotions and offer no healing. In order to take advantage of the respite from symptoms medications offer from intense emotional pain, use this time to dig deep and uproot the cause of the pain. The truth of the matter is that everything you have experienced still lives within you.

For PTSD sufferers, suppressing symptoms does not come close to helping them get to the other side of a traumatic experience. Denying and stifling symptoms of PTSD is not healthy. It is dangerous. Over time, a traumatic event or events will keep alive their triggers and thcy will awaken over and over and over until a change in dealing with the emotions, beliefs, and behaviors around them is addressed. You might believe that your life is now ruined and irreparable damage has been done because you believe you cannot 'get over it.' Brave military Veterans experience this as a normal part of returning home after war. The suicide rate among Veterans is 50% higher than that of civilians and those who have experienced a traumatic event are more likely to commit suicide than someone who hasn't. But PTSD and Complex PTSD can be helped.

As stated before, there are two forms of PTSD: Complex Post Traumatic Stress Disorder (CPTSD) and Post Traumatic Stress Disorder (PTSD). Complex Post Traumatic Stress Disorder is similar to the symptoms of PTSD but provokes a diagnosis built on long-term circumstances rather than a one time or briefly repeated incident. For those with Complex PTSD the painful circumstances are repeated over a long period of time such as a child who is exposed to repeated sexual abuse, domestic violence, enraged and controlling parents, frightening parental screaming, neglect, bullying, or some other emotionally and psychologically altering and painful experience. Each time the unwanted experience happens, it is equivalent to flicking the marbles over and over. Your emotional and psychological self keeps getting assaulted.

There are three ways your body/mind/spirit responds to trauma, no matter what the trauma is or how often it happens: 1. fight, 2. flight, or 3. freeze. Knowing how your body/mind/spirit reacted will help you better understand the wounds and symptoms that manifested. Everything is connected: thoughts>emotions>behavior. Realizations will unfold as you write.

PTSD and Complex PTSD are not your normal stress experiences. And they ought not be treated as such. These mental health conditions do not go away with a calming bath, a massage, or a day at the beach.

PTSD and Complex PTSD will not go away unaddressed but linger and remain a part of daily life. They will haunt you at unsuspecting moments, push you to depression or anxiety, anger or irritability, as well as a myriad of other symptoms making you feel powerless. PTSD and Complex PTSD are seriously disturbing. There is no doubt of this. Although Complex PTSD has not been added to the DSM-5 as its own disorder, Complex PTSD, in my work with clients, is the root of many mental health conditions, mental illnesses, and addictions.

Here are two lists to help you think about your wounds and their manifested symptoms. Refer to this list as you write through the weeks.

1. List of Wounds (*list not all inclusive*)

Loss of identity

Loss of security

Loss of comfort

Loss of belief you are safe

Loss of personal integrity

Loss of belief people are good

Loss of belief people are loyal

Loss of confidence

Loss of belief you are beautiful

Loss of belief you are lovable

Loss of belief you are wanted

Loss of belief you are worthy

Loss of memory of what really happened in the order it happened

Loss of trust

Loss of the power to have your own voice

Loss of personal value

Loss of purpose

Loss of meaning for life

Loss of faith

2. List of Symptoms (*list not all inclusive*)

Ways you and your body adapted or maladapted to wounds.

Being in a constant state of alarm

Feel tension

Feel frustration

Act recklessly

Sabotage your, or someone else's, happiness and/or success

Engage in wishes or actions of self-harm

Engage in suicidal attempts or thoughts of suicide

Emotionally shut down

Get depressed

Feel despair

Dissociate

Feel rage

Have uncontrollable impulses

Feel deep self-hate

Act out of a need to survive

Fear social events

Fear being vulnerable

Fear intimacy

Fear being exposed

Have poor concentration

Have fragmented thoughts

The writing course below has been effective in regulating PTSD responses to triggers, abating addictive behaviors, enabling a sense of wholeness, and planning for a bright future. For those who wrote through this writing course, dysphoric mood decreased and when traumatic memories arose physiological responses of depression or anxiety were reduced or disappeared. The recovery process was imbibed with hope and empowerment because facing emotions about what happened and working through this process freed up toxic emotions calming the body, mind and spirit.

In this journal you will find questions to help you recover from your PTSD or Complex PTSD. I recommend that you write these questions with pen and paper and not type them on a device. Studies show that writing changes the brain because it uses a different part of the brain than typing.

In an article by graphologist Seifer, he mentions the following benefits to writing:

1. calms the brain,
2. writing in cursive coordinates the left and right brain,
3. boosts cognitive skills,
4. inspires creativity,
5. sharpens the aging mind,
6. improves memory, and
7. uses more of your brain, and
8. has a lasting effect on memory.

Science is still out on all the abilities one's brain has to heal. As a witness to my own healing, and that of my clients, I can say without a doubt that writing is a powerful and effective way to recover from seemingly powerless and unresolvable traumatic experiences.

It is best to work through the following six stages of the 6-week writing course, *Unveil The Wounded Self*, with therapeutic help, just in case writing these steps brings up more than you can understand on your own. When going through this process, work with a professional counselor and make sure the counselor is well versed in PTSD and Complex PTSD, not just life's usual stressful situations. They are not the same. Please do not feel shame about this. No one should ever handle PTSD or Complex PTSD without a sounding board. NO ONE! Talk about your trauma, write about your trauma, know what has changed you and believe that you can recover. There is hope!

Here is the outline for the six-week course. I recommend that each item be given at least one week to process so you have time to think, assess, and assimilate the inner work you are doing. Respect the process. Respect yourself.

1. Write, in detail, what happened—(you walked into an alley, it was dank, dark, a hand grabbed your neck…) In other words—write JUST THE FACTS! If you have symptoms from Complex PTSD, choose an event or one repetitive incident to start. It is impossible to cover a whole life in one writing.
2. Write your experience of what happened—(the alley was dank, dark, and your stomach squeezed because you sensed danger, you proceeded nervously, a hand grabbed you, you thought, Oh God, he's going to kill me…) This step includes your inner experience.
3. Write the wounds inflicted upon you from what happened and the way you behave around these wounds. There are two parts to internal wounds: 1. the wound itself e.g. loss of innocence from being sexually abused, fear of vulnerability, fear of trusting and 2. your reaction to the wound, e.g., you avoid sex or you lie in order to ward off someone's anger, you stay suspicious of others, or you don't share emotions so as to not be vulnerable,

you blame others before they focus on you to avoid shame. This step is the heart of the course. Make sure you write both aspects in full detail. This step helps you acknowledge and get to the root of the PTSD. The root is not your fault. But you do not have to remain a victim.

4. Write what your wounds need in order to recover—(a better body image, willingness to trust yourself, willingness to trust others, to start dating again, take a class, go away for a weekend alone, speak up about your emotions, contact old friends) What do your wounds need in order to heal? How do you want to change your behaviors?
5. Write your healed vision of yourself and your life. You have dreams of what you want your life to look and feel like—(you envision living a life of joy with good friends, living by the beach or in the woods, have full trust in yourself, buy sexy things without fear, talk to authority without insecurity, teach a class, exercise). Cut out pictures from magazines that give you the feeling you want for your life. Paste them on a poster board to create a vision board. Use only those pictures that feel like the life you want. Put your collage in a place where you can study it daily.
6. Write what you are willing to do in order to create this healthy life on your vision board. Make a plan for wanted changes in your thoughts/beliefs>emotions>and behavior (forgive yourself, approach decisions with confidence, confront your fears, continue journal writing, join a support group, list new beliefs about life, list new beliefs about yourself, eat healthier, exercise, talk to a counselor, take up painting) Make the list as succinct as possible. Adjust them on a regular basis as you make progress to keep focused on a wellness plan. This is not complicated. It is as easy as writing a grocery list. It will even become enjoyable and satisfying.

Ideas to Calm Your Nervous System

To awaken, to open up
like a flower to the light of a fuller consciousness!
I want to see and feel and expand...

—Emily Carr

from *Hundreds and Thousands: The Journals of an Artist*

This list provides some of the ways in which you can calm your nervous system if your emotions get agitated while writing. Please do not abandon the process if you get anxious or depressed. These ideas will help so you can continue the writing process.

1. TAT (Tappas Acupuncture Treatment)

See: http://www.tatlife.com/ Acupressure Position for TAT:

Take your thumb and ring finger and place them on either side of the top of your nose—under your eyebrows above the tear ducts. Place your middle finger on your third eye. Take your other hand and gently cup the bottom of your skull at the back of your head. This exercise should be done no longer than 4 minutes. All you need to do while holding this position is to focus on the pained feeling you don't want. There is a free manual on this technique that you can download on the website mentioned above.

2. Emotional Freedom Technique (EFT)

Google for the best explanation of this healing process.

3. Faster Emotional Freedom Technique (EFT)

Google FAST EFT for a quicker tapping process.

4. Tips to calm the nervous system:

a. drink cool water—avoid the cold water that can make the nervous system contract,

b. drink warm tea,

c. sit in a hot to warm bath,

d. meditate while visualizing your nervous system relaxing,

e. stop writing—do something else,

f. wash your hands and face in cool water,

g. eat something clean like a bowl of organic strawberries, peaches, apples, papaya,

h. walk leisurely focusing on each step and take a few deep breaths,

i. take Vitamin C—eat an orange, ½ glass of orange juice, parsley tea (fresh, not tea bag). Take a handful of fresh parsley and drop it into a pot of boiling water,

j. read something inspiring,

k. take a few drops of Rescue Remedy, a wonderful tincture for calming the system,

l. take Vitamin B,

m. get a gentle full-body massage,

n. give yourself a foot massage,

o. give yourself an ear massage,

p. do yoga—the downward dog series is fabulous, or

q. do tai chi—the graceful and gentle movements can help you feel light and flowing.

Six Week Writing Course

To write is to descend, to excavate, to go underground.

—Anais Nin

from *The Diary of Anais Nin, Volume Five, 1947-1955*

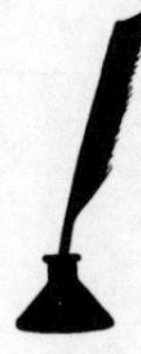

WEEK ONE

What Happened?

The truth about childhood is stored up in our body and lives in the depth of our soul. Our intellect can be deceived, our feelings can be numbed and manipulated, our perception shamed and confused, our bodies tricked with medication. But our soul never forgets. And because we are one, one whole soul in one body, someday our body will present its bill.

—Alice Miller
from *Rage to Courage*

Write what happened to you. Write just the facts! Was it one event, such as 9-11 or a deployment into a war zone, or a repeated event, such as the effects of being neglected by an alcoholic parent, being sexual abused over the course of years, growing up poor, given hurtful comments about who you are. You can choose whatever memory holds the most emotional or psychological distress. Start there!

WEEK TWO

What is Your Experience of What Happened?

Clutter and mess show us that life is being lived... Tidiness makes me think of held breath, of suspended animation... Perfectionism is a mean, frozen form of idealism, while messes are the artist's true friend. What people somehow forgot to mention when we were children was that we need to make messes in order to find out who we are and why we are here.

—Anne Lamott

Write your personal inner experience of what happened. This is your inner narrative story that no one knows but you. Write what you saw, heard, tasted, touched. Write about any sensations, thoughts, beliefs, or any other inner experience you had. Write in as much detail as possible. This is where you simply pour it all out.

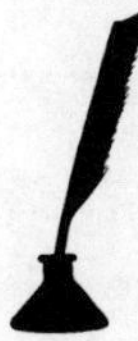

WEEK THREE

What Wounds Did You Incur from What Happened?

Storytelling is healing. As we reveal ourselves in story, we become aware of the continuing core of our lives under the fragmented surface of our experience. We become aware of the multifaceted, multi-chaptered 'I' who is the storyteller. We can trace out the paradoxical and even contradictory versions of ourselves that we create for different occasions, different audiences… Most important, as we become aware of ourselves as storytellers, we realize that what we understand and imagine about ourselves is a story. And when we know all this, we can use our stories to heal and make ourselves whole.

—Susan Wittig Albert
from *Writing From Life: Telling Your Soul's Story*

This is a crucial step. Write, in detail, the unwanted feelings, thoughts, and behaviors that resulted from the moment of the traumatic event or events. These unwanted changes incurred deep inner wounds. They changed you. These wounds always involve internal losses. Write the ways in which your behaviors changed since the painful and traumatic event or events. The root of a wound has to do with the internal losses or unwanted changes. Symptoms are how you behaviorally maladapted.

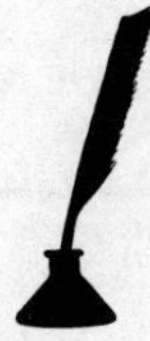

WEEK FOUR

What Do Your Wounds Need?

If I do not write to empty my mind, I go mad.

—George Gordon Byron

from *Hours Of Idleness*

Wounds always need something for healing. When you have a physical injury it is easy to see what you need. It can be more difficult to assess inner wounds. But you do have needs and desires around them and that makes it easier for wounds to be identified. Refer to your list of wounds in the previous week and write what each wound needs in order to recover.

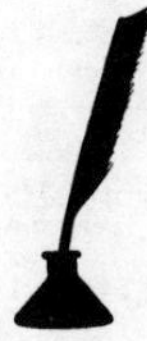

WEEK FIVE

Make a Vision of Your Healed Self and Life

People do not 'have' diseases, which are really descriptive mechanisms created by contemporary medicine. People have stories, and the stories are narratives of their lives, their relationships, and the way they experience an illness. .

—Arthur Kleinman

from *The Illness Narratives - Suffering, Healing and the Human Condition*

Collect magazine pictures, photos or draw your own, that resemble what you imagine your recovered self and life to look like. Paste them on a poster board. You can add words anywhere you want on the board. Be creative. By holding a vision of your recovered self and life and by having something to look at, you begin to set an internal vision for your recovery. On this page write your new narrative, the one you want to create for yourself. Most libraries have a table of free magazines. The good thing about this chart is that you can add whatever you want, or remove what you don't.

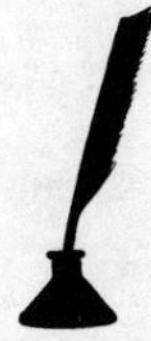

WEEK SIX

Write out a future plan for wellness

Write the vision: make it plain on tablets…
for still the vision awaits its appointed time…
—Habakkuk 2:2

Write out your plan for the future. What are you willing to do on a daily basis to keep yourself focused and moving forward? A plan should involve new beliefs and new behaviors. Review the plan once a month and change it according to what you still need to accomplish. When writing the new beliefs, write them by using causative and transformative words, phrases, and sentences that indicate changes from old dysfunctional beliefs to new ones. For example, you might say that your first plan is to speak up when you are angry. Include the changed belief: *I now believe* that I can let someone know when I am angry at them. The words "I now believe" are transformative words because they have taken an old belief and rephrased it into a new and healthier one. Another example is: *I now see* that to drink when I'm afraid is not the best way to deal with my fear. This rephrasing changes our brain through new language. As a result, we will have a healthier emotional reaction, and behave differently as well.

Uniting the Child with the Adult Self

~ A Writing Exercise ~

In the diary I could reestablish the balance.
Here I could be depressed, angry, disparaging, discouraged.
I could let out my demons.

—Anais Nin
from *The Measure of My Days*

In addition to the above writing program, this writing exercise will help you create the needed distance between memory and its psychic pain. The imagination is powerful and can be implemented whenever you need to call on it for emotional stability. This exercise works well with Complex PTSD.

All of us have two selves. One is the public persona and the other the private authentic self that only we know. When we write we get to drop into the authentic self which helps us regulate our public self.

Step 1

With your dominant hand write out a detailed situation from the past that continues to be painful. This step is to be written from the perspective of the adult point of view as you remember it. Make sure to include all the senses that were involved. Take as long as it takes until you have written the full story. Do not stress about grammar. Write in a stream-of-consciousness, free-write style and just let your experience of this story spill out onto the page. Again, this is to be written from the adult point of view.

Step 2

With your non-dominant hand write out the same story in detail from the child's point of view, again, including all the senses. Do not shift to your dominant hand just because it might be easier. The point of using your non-dominant hand is to replicate the sense of vulnerability that a child feels in painful situations. Again, use the stream-of-consciousness, free-write form. Do not concern yourself with grammar. Just write the situation from the child's point of view and get the full story onto the page. Use a colored pencil or crayon if it will help you stay in the child's point of view.

Step 3

With your dominant hand write out how you wished the situation had happened. Again write this step in the stream-of-consciousness, free-write style.

Purpose

The purpose of writing from the point of view in Step 3, is to bring together the fragmented and injured parts of yourself into a healed picture. Although this exercise usually has healing benefits in only one writing, some people write the memory out several times until they feel pain release and let go. The process is unique for each person. We can rewrite our narrative for a powerful change. Our perspective shifts inside us when we invent our own endings to painful situations or change the point of view from adult to child. Getting psychological distance from our usual perspective allows emotional pain to heal. Try it!

AGE EVENT CHART

Here is a chart to help you organize traumatic events in your life into a series of age groups. Feel free to change the headings if needed.

Age	Physical	Emotional	Health	Family	Strangers	Jobs	Money
Age 3-8							
Age 8-12							

Age	Physical	Emotional	Health	Family	Strangers	Jobs	Money
Age 13-18							
Age 18-25							
Age 26-35							

Age	Physical	Emotional	Health	Family	Strangers	Jobs	Money
Age 36-40							
Age 41-45							
Age 46-50							

Age	Physical	Emotional	Health	Family	Strangers	Jobs	Money
Age 51-55							
Age 56-60							
Age 61-65							

Age	Physical	Emotional	Health	Family	Strangers	Jobs	Money
Age 65-70							
Age 70-75							

About the Author

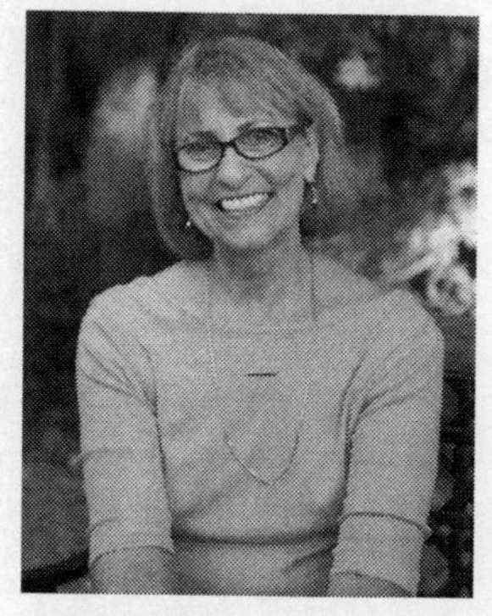

Jan Marquart, LCSW, author, has been writing in her daily journal since June, 1972 and has written more than one hundred journals. Through her own writing process, Jan has realized that daily writing has kept her life inspired and allowed her to heal her own PTSD. She teaches this writing process in her psychotherapy practice, Story Circle Network, and Life Learning Institute for people over fifty. She is the founder of a six-week writing program titled, *The Provocation of Journal Writing* as well as the six-week program titled, *Unveil the Wounded Self- Write to Heal PTSD.* Jan's books are on JanMarquart.com and CanYouFindMyLove.com. Her professional website is JanMarquartLCSW.wordpress.com.

NOTES

NOTES

NOTES

NOTES

Made in the USA
Middletown, DE
23 May 2018